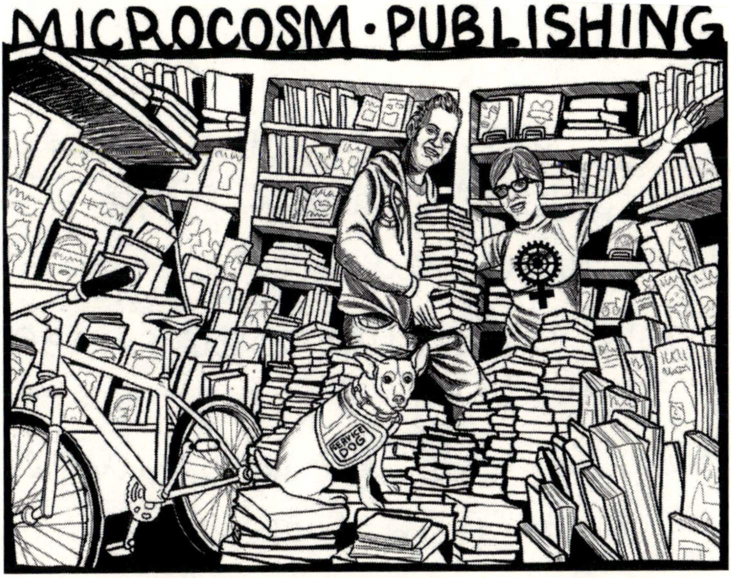


**MICROCOSM PUBLISHING** is Portland's most diversified publishing house and distributor, with a focus on the colorful, authentic, and empowering. Our books and zines have put your power in your hands since 1996, equipping readers to make positive changes in their lives and in the world around them. Microcosm emphasizes skill-building, showing hidden histories, and fostering creativity through challenging conventional publishing wisdom with books and bookettes about DIY skills, food, bicycling, gender, self-care, and social justice. What was once a distro and record label started by Joe Biel in a drafty bedroom was determined to be *Publishers Weekly*'s fastest-growing publisher of 2022 and #3 in 2023 and 2024, and is now among the oldest independent publishing houses in Portland, OR, and Cleveland, OH. We are a politically moderate, centrist publisher in a world that has inched to the right for the past 80 years.

# Table of Contents



— 2017 —

# why should SEX EDUCATORS be informed about disability

when it comes to sexuality, people with physical or intellectual disabilities are often seen as asexual or hypersexual. their sexuality is heavily regulated and/or seen as dangerous or inappropriate. in reality:

IT IS NOT INAPPROPRIATE FOR INTELLECTUALLY OR PHYSICALLY DISABLED FOLKS TO DESIRE OR ENGAGE IN SEXUAL ACTIVITIES.

this zine is an introduction to some thinkers/artists/activists and their ideas & concepts that deal with the intersection of disability & sexuality!

# let's begin*

with an overview of some important and foundational concepts & terms used in both the academic & activist communities. there is a lot of overlap with intersectional feminist ideas/concepts, which are also an important area of study for sex educators (and all other humans). for more info on intersectional feminism in general, check out people like Kimberlé Crenshaw, bell hooks, Audre Lorde, Gloria Anzaldua & Roxanne Gay

# concepts & terms

**medical model of disability**

the idea that the disabled body is in some way "broken" and needs to be fixed / cured

**social model of disability**

the disability is created by physical and social structures, and is problematic for the disabled person not because their body / mind is broken, but because the physical / cultural structure does not take their body's / mind's needs into account

**temporarily able-bodied (TAB)**

a term that is used to both describe people without a disability and also call attention to the reality that this is a fluid state and could change (accidents, old age, etc.)

intersectionality

the way that multiple identities (ie: disabled, black, straight, middle-class) interact to create oppressions & privileges (this can shift based on the context & culture)

ableism

the valuing of people who are TAB over those with physical or mental disabilities. like racism, sexism, classism, etc., ableism creates a hierarchy and gives privileges to some, while oppressing others.

compulsory able-bodiedness

the (often unconscious) assumption that not having a disability is the "natural" or "normal" state of being (compared to Adrienne Rich's concept of "compulsory heterosexuality")

# self

by Adina K. Burke

You are allergic to latex. That is why your cooch feels like a portal to hell. Please see your doctor as soon as possible, do not assume that this is "what it's supposed to feel like."

Sex Ed failed you.

Pillows offer great leverage, use them.

Even when sitting down your ass is still smackable.

He will break your heart. Let him. It will be a good lesson.

Just because she has a clit doesn't mean she knows what to do with yours. Speak up.

Invest in yourself. Buy a nice toy.

Laughing in that doctor's face when they questioned your sexual activity level was the right thing to do, even though others said differently.

Use lube. Please.

Clothing pins and nipple clamps are totally not the same thing.

Do not stand for mediocre love. Do not stand for a shitty fuck.

If one admires your body, it does not mean they are admiring you. Give yourself time to learn this. Let go.

Let it go. You are more than your body. You are the trembling of tongues and the mess of the sheets, long red hair in the shower drain, forgotten toothbrush, mispronounced name of the night

And sometimes you are not. And that is okay.

before diving in to the intersection of

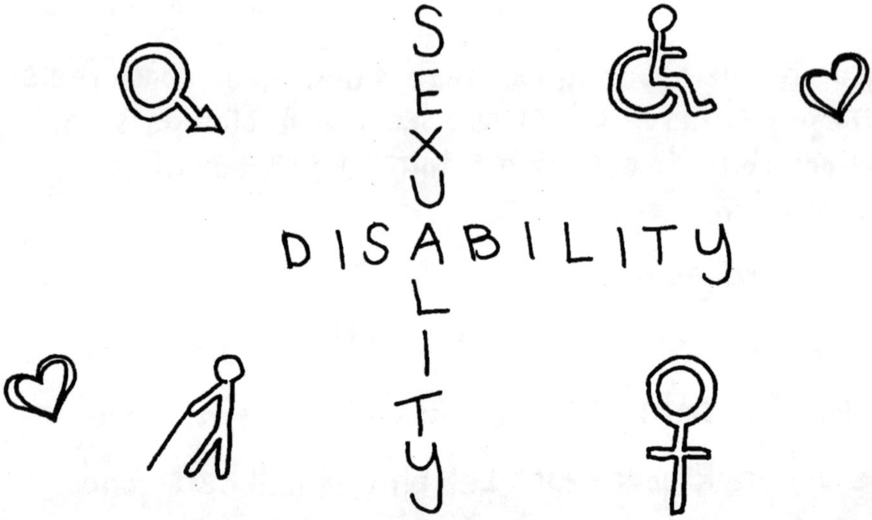


let's take a look at the concept of

# disability justice

as defined by Patty Berne on the website sinsinvalid.org. the 10 principles include:

1. intersectionality
2. leadership of the most impacted
3. anti-capitalist
4. commitment to cross movement organizing
5. recognizing wholeness
6. sustainability
7. cross-disability solidarity
8. interdependenc
9. collective acces
10. collective liberatio

additionally, patty writes:

“a disability justice framework understands that all bodies are unique & essential, that all bodies have strengths & needs that must be met. we know that we are powerful not despite the complexities of our bodies, but because of them. we understand that all bodies are caught in these bindings of ability, race, gender, sexuality, class, nation state and imperialism, and that we cannot separate them. these are the positions from which we struggle.”

# how to talk to a new lover about cerebral palsy by eli clare

tell her: complete strangers
have patted my head, kissed
my cheek, called me courageous.

tell this story more than once, ask
her to hold you, rock you
against her body, breast to back,

her arms curving round, only
you flinch unchosen, right arm trembles
don't use the word *spastic*.

in europe after centuries
of death by exposure
and drowning,
they banished us
to the streets

let her feel the tension burn down your arms,
tremors jump. take it slow: when she asks
about the difference between CP and MS,

refrain from handing her an encyclopedia.
if you leave, know that you will ache.
resist the urge to ignore your body. tell her:

they taunted me retard, monkey,
defect. the words sank into my body.
the rocks and fists left bruises.

gimps and crips, caps
in hand, we still
wander the streets but now
the options abound: telethons,
nursing homes, welfare lines.

try not to be ashamed as you flinch and tremble
under her warm hands. think of the stories you haven't
told yet. tension locks behind your shoulder blades.

ask her what she thinks as your hands shake
along her body, sleep curled against her,
and remember to listen: she might surprise you.

from the marrow's telling:
words in motion

# Working with the *body*

it's important to remember the

— BODY —

when working with disability & sexuality.

You may want to check in about any shame or guilt experienced around the body.

You may also want to do interactive activities (like this!) ⟶ to promote acceptance & education. Not everyone understands what parts they have and what those parts do!

# my body

draw a picture of your external sex organs using the parts below as a guide, depending on what you have or don't have:

- vulva
- mons pubus
- clitoris
- vaginal lips (inner/outer)
- urethra
- introitus (vaginal opening)
- perineum
- bartholins glands
- penis
- testes
- scrotum
- anus
- pubic hair

an alternative way of looking at *sexuality* that could be helpful for disabled folks is making the distinction between a

# "Sex life" and ⟹

the assumption that an individual "has" sex, is able to control it, own it, & create a completely private, "particular and limited part of life" for it

Sex & Disability p. 39

must be "healthy", always looking for "better" sex or "the ultimate pleasure", often described as people "working on" their sex life.

Sex & Disability p. 42

occurs in the same types of places: bedrooms, hotels, baths, etc. (ie: private, owned or paid for in some way, not always accessible to all.)

ABLEIST

"when disability is linked to sex, it becomes a clinical matter in which each disability betrays a particular limitation of sexual opportunity, growth, or feeling." Sex & Disability p. 42

# Sexual Culture

(as defined & discussed by Tobin Siebers in "A Sexual Culture for Disabled People.")

- "... disability [is] not a defect that needs to be overcome to have sex, but a complex embodiment that enhances sexual activities and pleasure." Sex & Disability p.47
- POLITICAL → people w/ disabilities are SEXUAL CITIZENS.
- less focus on penetrative sex / sex with a beginning, middle, end — instead, there is an openness to eroticizing "non-typical" parts of the body & alternative sexual narratives (planned, different or no orgasms, alternative private spaces, etc.)

by opening up our definitions of sex & sexuality we can create more room for all types of people & bodies & relationships & identities

# Sex Toys

...and adapting them for different bodies (from the Ultimate Guide to Sex & Disability)

mobility & motor control:

- wearing a vibrator or toy on the body (around the waist to sit on the clitoris or around the penis) so you don't need to hold it
- remote control toys
- harnesses to hold a dildo in place on a partner or on a bed/wall, etc.

fatigue

- timing sex around medication or energy levels that fluxuate
- pillows or other props to hold you up so you don't have to

decreased sensation

- exploring all parts of the body to see what is enjoyable
- vibrators, paddles, whips, and floggers can create more pressure (but also be careful & know your limits)

increased sensation

- vibrators may be too much, so a non-vibrating toy might be better
- soft items like paint brushes or feathers can be enjoyable and inexpensive

privacy

- keep in consideration the accessibility and the noise of your toys (although music or TV could help mask the sound)
- soft rubber vibrators are the most quiet option
- ease of cleaning the toy is also important — water proof options are the simplest and quickest

we tend to think of

the erotic

as an easy, tantalizing

sexual arousal.

I speak of the erotic

as the deepest life force,

a force which moves us

toward living in a FUNDAMENTAL WAY.

and when I say LIVING I mean it as

that force which moves

us toward what will

accomplish REAL, POSITIVE

CHANGE. — Audre Lorde

# RESOURCES

- ♡ www.sexualityanddisability.org
- ♡ The Ultimate Guide to Sex and Disability: For All of Us Who Live with Disabilities, Chronic Pain, and Illness
  by Miranda Kaufman, Cory Silverberg, and Fran Odette
- ♡ Already Doing It
  by Michael Gill
- ♡ Sex and Disability
  edited by Robert McRuer and Anna Mollow
- ♡ The Marrow's Telling: Words in Motion
  by Eli Clare
- ♡ sinsinvalid.org
- ♡ PleasureABLE: Sexual Device Manual for Persons with Disabilities
  by Kate Naphtali, Edith MacHattie & Stacy Elliot